Elton,

To your health

:)

Kathleen

"Dr. Kathleen Carson is my go-to TMJ and sleep specialist on the West Coast. She has integrated a wealth of knowledge on airway, pain, sleep, and breathing."
M. Gelb, DMD; The Gelb Center

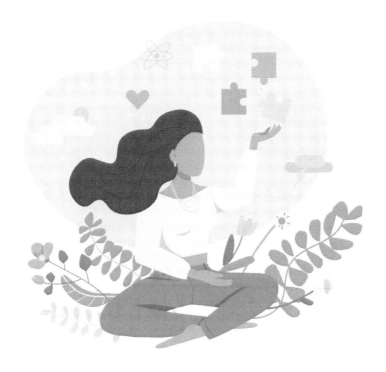

Introduction

——

This is a book to help those wanting to get better by offering tools and techniques to help themselves. As a dentist who treats chronic pain, TMJ, sleep disordered breathing and all the traditional dental issues—I have seen one thing we need to emphasize more. I have discovered how *you* can help yourself and as a result see vastly improved health.

As a practitioner, I have tools that I can use. However, there is no magic wand that will cure what causes anything that I treat.

My tools are just Band-Aids.

They are crutches designed to help relieve ***symptoms***. However, symptoms are just indicators of a much larger problem.

Much like the medications we provide for patients who have high blood pressure or sleeping difficulties, chronic pain, or almost any of modern societies health problems—my tools can help to ease symptoms.

To address the underlying issues, we need to turn our focus to the CAUSE—an underlying problem that results in the visible symptoms of disease.

Most of what you are being given to treat symptoms will only help you get by and survive — not thrive.

I want you to *thrive*.

There are no one size fits all answers. Each person is unique in what will best help them. However, there are some very significant universal patterns that apply to many situations.

If *you* want to *thrive*—we begin with a simple idea that *you* and *you* alone—hold the key, to once and for all correct the underlying cause of your dis-ease.

You will have to put in some work.

There are a multitude of tools out there to help relieve symptoms and that is important. These tools can be very effective. However, none of them will solve the underlying cause without work being done by YOU.

It begins with education. This book will provide the education. By educating yourself, you will be ready to begin doing the work. This book will introduce a variety of techniques you can use to eliminate pain, illness, and poor sleep cycles. Together, we will work to identify, address, and ultimately correct the underlying causes.

That is what this book is for. Within these pages—you learn a variety of ways *you* can help yourself.

This is not an all-inclusive, exhaustive manual and your learning will likely continue beyond this book. I will introduce you to many areas that are mandatory for you to get better. There are no short cuts.

Remember, there is no magic potion, magic appliance, or magic injection. *You are the magic.*

Modern medicine may help to relieve symptoms, but *you* have the power to address the underlying cause.

This does not mean that intervention from a doctor, a dentist, a wellness coach, an oral appliance, a technique, or medications should NOT be used—these will likely be necessary to help aid you in your journey to wellness.

It is possible that too much damage has been done. Your journey to health and wellness may require a combination of modern medical or dental intervention. Just remember, without the additional work that you will be required to do to achieve the outcome you want, these interventions will only relieve the symptoms and not eliminate the underlying cause. If you choose not to do the work, you will not only be selling yourself short—you will almost guarantee that additional problems will be a part of your life in the future.

As we begin our journey together, I will be introducing you to concepts that you have likely never thought about. I will introduce you to the important health benefits of effective *nasal breathing.* I will demonstrate how important it is to breathe correctly. You will learn how to breathe properly by using breathing exercises and techniques.

Healthy breathing is the first key to optimal health.

Proper and effective breathing will lead to significant improvement of your overall health and it will work to reduce, if not eliminate, symptoms of chronic health problems.

It is simple really. Breathe well to be well. You cannot expect to experience lasting improvement without proper breathing. Period. No exceptions. Once you have achieved the ability to properly breathe, you will then be ready to apply the other self-help concepts introduced in this book. Proper breathing applies universally to all of us. Once you are breathing correctly, your next step will be to learn what you, your mind and your body need to restore complete health. It will be your job to figure out which of the other principles and techniques you will need to address your individual needs.

Try them all. Apply them all. They will not be difficult. Try them one at a time or all together—that is up to you. If you are breathing properly—you will begin to see the benefits.

I have asked my colleague and good friend, Timbrey Lind, to contribute her expertise to this work. Timbrey is a hygienist, a myofunctional therapist, and a Buteyko breathing practitioner.

She educates individuals on how to better breathe, function, and lead a healthier life.

More information on her and what she provides can be found on her website www.integrativehygienist.com.

You will see her contributions as her name will appear below the titles of her contributions.

I will cite books and resources throughout where I have found valuable information and that you might want to use for further exploration.

Keep in mind that since this publication, there are likely additional topics to cover and possibly changes to the information presented here. Ask your doctors and other health care providers for their expertise as well.

Nasal Breathing

—

You must breathe through your nose. End of
story. If you cannot, you must change that.
This chapter will cover the whys and the hows
so that you can achieve this. It is step one. It is
NOT optional. Nothing else will make a lasting
impact if you cannot achieve this primary goal.

Proper breathing is medicine - ancient practices
knew this, we somehow forgot it. Possibly
because we cannot patent it, we cannot bottle it,
and no big company is making money on it. It
did not fit into "modern medicine" as no one
was paying for it to be taught or practiced.
Today, this is starting to change as we are all
starting to wake up and realize how we are being
manipulated in marketing, education, social
media, almost everything we are exposed to
these days has underlying manipulation

carefully designed to sway what we do, what we buy, how we look, and what we think.

Health care is no exception. As a player in the health care arena, over the years I have become absolutely horrified by how little is done to help patients be able to prevent the need for our services and how much is done to keep them hooked on the things that are sold and used to treat symptoms. All too often, we are only treating disease, not promoting wellness. This is one of the best kept secrets out there. It is something that FINALLY my profession is acknowledging, and we are hearing more and more about it. Yet, every single day I come across someone who has NO IDEA and cannot believe they have never been told this. Which tells me that even though it appears that in my little circle of the big world huge progress is being made, it has not reached the critical tipping point where it is easily found as common knowledge. I would like to change that.

Breathing is one of the most powerful things we have control over that can impact multiple areas of our health. It is often overlooked. It affects every internal organ, our heart rate, our digestion, our sleep, our moods, our athletic performance, our autonomic nervous system - nothing goes untouched by how we breathe.

Every breath has the potential to have either a positive or a negative impact on our body.

Believe it or not, in research it has been well established that normal breathing should be through the nose more than 90% of the time. Ideally, 96% of the time. Some of us have been taught that in through the nose and out through the mouth is the best breath. I disagree. Exhaling through the nose results in more oxygen being delivered to the body more efficiently. Nasal breathing has been well documented to provide many health benefits.

The WHY's behind nasal breathing:

The nose is equipped with a complex filtering mechanism which purifies the air we breathe before it enters the lungs.

Human nasal passages are a built-in air purifier and humidifier that you do not get to take advantage of if you are not using it.

Our sinuses produce mucus which trap pathogens (the bad bugs) that enter our body. Cilia (tiny little hairs) line the nasal cavity, trapping the mucous and the bad bugs. The cilia then beat out this contaminated mucous for us to swallow and digest (and we also blow it out).

In addition, blood lines the nasal mucosa providing immune function by bringing immune cells to the area. These immune cells in the blood vessels of the nose can mount a systemic response earlier on than if you are breathing through the mouth. Breathing though your mouth bypasses this entire nasal immune system.

NITRIC OXIDE (NO)

One of the most important reasons for nasal breathing is the production of nitric oxide. Nitric Oxide is produced in our nasal cavities and we can absorb up to six times more nitric oxide by breathing through our nose. Nitric Oxide is believed to play a vital role in many biological events including regulation of blood flow, platelet function, immunity, and neurotransmission. Nitric oxide enhances the lungs capacity to absorb oxygen – we can, on average, absorb 18% more oxygen with nasal breathing compared to mouth breathing. It turns out the best oxygen exchange, the most blood perfusion in the lungs, is in the lower lobes of the lungs. Nitric oxide allows the oxygen to be taken lower in the lungs and allow for better oxygen exchange. If we are breathing through our mouths, only our upper lungs (chest breathing) and not lower lungs (diaphragmatic breathing) is occurring. There is not enough time or depth in the lungs for good O2 exchange to take place.

THE AUTONOMIC NERVOUS SYSTEM

Stanford Medical School discovered there is a pacemaker in your brain that monitors your breathing. If you breathe fast, that pacemaker sends signals of agitation to your brain. When we are breathing through our mouth, we are mainly ventilating the upper chest. It is believed by breathing experts that most of us are chronically breathing faster and taking in more air than we need, typically through the mouth. This stimulates a fight or flight response in the body which means that the sympathetic nervous system is activated, and stress hormones are being produced. Over time, our body acclimates to this and it feels "normal" though your system is constantly in a level of sympathetic stress resulting in too much cortisol (stress hormone) being constantly released leading to what has been called "adrenal fatigue". Mouth breathing = Chest breathing = fast = fight or flight = stressed = sympathetic nervous system. You cannot establish diaphragmatic breathing if you are mouth breathing. We will discuss the importance of this later.

Nose breathing, on the other hand, slows down the breath. Long slow breaths are relaxing. Nasal breathing carries the air deeper into the lungs (nitric oxide) and activates the diaphragm. A typical adult engages as little as 10% of the range of the diaphragm when breathing, which overburdens the heart, elevates blood pressure, and causes circulatory problems. Studies show that extending those breaths to 50-70% of the diaphragm's capacity will ease cardiovascular stress and allow the body to work more efficiently. Diaphragmatic breathing reduces heart rates, increases insulin, reduces glycemia, reduces free radical production, increases antioxidant status, decreases cortisol, and increases melatonin.

This is the result of activating the parasympathetic nervous system (relaxation). Slow, nasal, diaphragmatic breathing stimulates the vagus nerve, opening communication along the vagal network, and relaxes us into a parasympathetic state. This is the best way we can take control over our chronically hyperactive sympathetic nervous system and stressed-out states. It all starts with calm, slow, deep, nasal breathing.

Restorative breathing techniques have been practiced in Hinduism, Buddhism, Christianity, and other religions for thousands of years. Science has only recently caught up and shown how they can reduce blood pressure, boost athletic performance, and balance the nervous system.

Today, it is estimated that 15% of the American population suffer from an autoimmune disorder - when our immune system goes rogue and attacks healthy tissues. Many of these autoimmune disorders are tied to dysfunction of the autonomic nervous system. Proper breathing can help rebalance the system, heal the body, and rewire the mind. Proper breathing should be part of all comprehensive treatment plans.

ATHLETIC PERFORMANCE & WEIGHT LOSS

The athletic benefits of nasal breathing are many. It helps improve endurance, allows for shorter recovery times, and maintains hydration. Nasal breathing helps ensure we are mostly exercising in the optimal aerobic zone, whereas if you are predominately mouth breathing you are in the anaerobic zone.

Breathing through your nose can cut total exertion in half. When we run our cells aerobically with oxygen, we gain 16x more energy efficiency over anaerobic. In fact, breathing less during exercise creates a lower oxygen environment which can mimic training at altitude and over time your body adapts, and improved mitochondrial function and increased red blood cell production can occur. In addition, breathing through the nose helps us to maintain hydration; mouth breathing causes the body to lose 40% more water.

70% of the US population is considered overweight. 1 in 3 of us is obese. Neither exercise nor diet alone will help you lose weight in a healthy way. Have you ever wondered where the fat goes? If you are like most of us, you probably think most fat is excreted through bodily fluids. It is not.

Based on the research from the British Medical Journal, most fat turns into carbon dioxide which is exhaled when we breathe (Meerman & Brown, 2014).

Fat loss starts with nasal breathing. Good health starts with nasal breathing. Better performance starts with nasal breathing.

The lungs are the weight regulating system of the body. For every 10 lbs. of fat lost, 8.5lbs come out through the lungs - mostly carbon dioxide mixed with water. The rest is sweated or urinated out. Proper gas exchange, and breathing habits, are necessary for proper weight regulation.

Most of our clients are living in a stressed state (or the sympathetic branch of our nervous system). Not only is this the sugar burning system, but it also leads to abnormally high levels of cortisol. High cortisol levels promote weight gain (Sominsky & Spencer, 2014).

The more oxygen our bodies use, the more fat we will burn. Fats are large molecules made up of oxygen, carbon, and hydrogen. When the oxygen we breathe reaches these fat molecules, it breaks them down into carbon dioxide and water. The blood then picks up the carbon dioxide – a waste product of our bodies – and returns it to the lungs to be exhaled. Nasal breathing is more efficient than mouth breathing in terms of supplying oxygen to the body as well as the transfer of oxygen and carbon dioxide between the lungs and red blood cells. (more Nitric Oxide in slower nasal breathing = carried lower in the lungs = better O2 exchange) When performing cardiovascular exercise, it is therefore preferable to inhale and exhale through the nose (*Novotny, 2007*).

BETTER POSTURE

Who does not want better posture? It is estimated that about half of the population suffers from poor posture that results in compromised health. Poor posture can be a result of an inadequate airway. Think of it as unconsciously putting yourself in the CPR position to allow better airflow - head up, neck tilted, chin out - easier air passage in what otherwise might be a compromised airway. It goes the other way as well though…. Studies have shown that breathing through the mouth can modify the head position, regardless of if you are compensating or not. Children with nasal breathing, age 8 and above, present with better posture than those with continued mouth breathing beyond age 8 and that this continues into adulthood. The result is decreased muscle strength, reduced chest expansion, and impaired lung ventilation. It also effects respiratory mechanics and exercise capacity. Not only are you breathing worse, but the resulting postural changes increases the weight of our head - for every inch of forward head posture, the weight of the head increases by an additional 10 lbs.

Therefore, with a forward head posture of two inches (which is quite common), the average twelve-pound head now weighs 34 pounds! For all you TMJ pain patients, this means increased stress on your muscles, headaches more easily triggered, neck pain, TMJ tension, spinal issues…. The list goes on and on. Poor breathing habits lead to poor breathing results and decreased quality of life if not corrected.

SLEEP

Nasal breathing benefits do not just occur during waking hours. When breathing and oxygenation are even subtly compromised during sleep, it increases your body's stress response. Nasal congestion can worsen subjective sleep quality and can be a major challenge for the treatment of Sleep Disordered Breathing (SDB). By treating nasal obstruction, we can improve sleep, make appliance use easier, and improve quality of life. Studies show that nasal congestion is strongly associated with snoring, restless sleep, and excessive daytime sleepiness. This can be a result of disrupted or poor-quality sleep cycles, reduced oxygen delivery, increased sympathetic responses, or several other issues that develop while we are not breathing through our nose at night. It may or may not be accompanied by snoring, I have treated numerous "non-snorers" who have sleep issues because of not breathing in a healthy way at night.

Speaking of snoring, no amount of snoring is normal. No amount of sleep disordered breathing comes without risks of serious health effects. Dr. Guilleminault (sleep researcher at Stanford) found that in children who showed only heavy breathing and light snoring or increased respiratory effort—could suffer from mood disorders, blood pressure derangements, learning disabilities, and more.

Snoring is almost three times more likely in children with chronic rhinitis and they are more than five times more likely to suffer from sleep disruption compared to those without the runny noses. When seasonal allergies hit, incidences of sleep apnea and breathing difficulties rise. The nose gets stuffed, we start mouth breathing, and the airways collapse. Sleeping with an open mouth exacerbates these problems. Gravity pulls the soft tissues in the throat and tongue down, closing off the airway even more.

A report from the Mayo Clinic found that chronic insomnia, long assumed to be a psychological problem, is often a breathing problem. You cannot sleep because you cannot breathe.

Mouth taping at night is growing in popularity because the benefits of nasal breathing at night allows a much more calm, deep, and restorative sleep. We will get into this topic in the next section.

The oral mucosa is not capable of an adequate amount of humidification. An easy way to determine if someone is mouth breathing in their sleep is to ask if their mouth is dry in the morning or if they need water at their bedside.

MOUTH HEALTH

Mouth breathing contributes to periodontal disease, bad breath, and is the number one cause of cavities - even more damaging than sugar consumption, poor diet, or poor hygiene.

Mouth breathing directly affects dental health by causing the drying of oral structures and the decrease of saliva production. It also causes a decrease in the pH of the mouth (more acidic) which allows the bad bugs to thrive. Saliva acts to neutralize acid in the mouth and helps to flush away bacteria. Without saliva and its beneficial protective mechanisms, risk of decay and periodontal disease, the pathological inflammation of the gum and bone support surrounding the teeth, increases. During sleep, mouth breathing decreases intra oral pH as compared to normal breathing. This lowered pH can lead to erosion of tooth surfaces, increased sensitivity of the teeth to temperatures and susceptibility to tooth decay.

All those things' patients typically see the dentist for - by simply closing your mouth and breathing through your nose, your oral health will improve more than anything else you can do. You can floss all you want…. Your gum tissue will NOT be healthy if you are breathing through your mouth.

CHILDREN

This is not a book about our kids - but I would be remiss if I do not get back to my main point of SOLVING these issues before they become problems. Therefore, I am including a small section on why you should make sure your kids, your friends' kids, your grandkids, your neighbors' kids, all kids you come across who are not breathing through their noses. This ONE change in a kid's life can make a huge difference - and if all goes well, they might never realize the changed trajectory of their lives for the better.

If a kid is breathing predominately through their mouth, they are suffering all the consequences above in addition to other signs and symptoms that often go unrelated. I will cover just a few in hopes that it convinces you to intervene and stop this cycle.

There is now a plethora of evidence that children with sleep disordered breathing (SDB) show deficits in neurocognitive performance, behavioral impairments, and school performance. It has been shown that some of the neurocognitive consequences are reversible while others may be irreversible if left untreated early on. Behavioral impairments include (but are not limited to) ADHD, aggressive behavior, impulsivity, hyperactivity, and decreased attention. Did you know that sleep disordered breathing includes simply breathing through the mouth at night? I can almost guarantee you that if they are mouth breathing during the day, they are mouth breathing at night. AND just because they are not mouth breathing during the day, it does not mean it is the same at night.

Sleep fragmentation for these kids is thought to be a major culprit.

There is help there for the kids, and the earlier the better. If you would like more information on what this might include at various ages and stages (from a newborn on up), then just ask... we can help.

There is nothing complicated about nasal breathing. The first step is making sure you CAN breathe through your nose (next section) and then getting used to breathing through your nose with your mouth closed.

How to Improve Nasal Breathing
———

First thing first. CAN you breathe through your nose? There are three basic answers:

1. Yes, absolutely, and very comfortably you
   can sit with your lips closed and breathe

solely through your nose with little effort for any length of time.

2. Yes, kind of - but not comfortably or with extra effort or for a short time. Not consistently due to allergies & congestion fall in here too.

3. NO, not at all.

Let us start with group one - the yes, absolutely, group. AWESOME! Now my question is…. But do you do it ALL of the time - or at least 90% of the time? Most do not or do not know. Often, it is habit and just not realizing that is what your nose is for. You are supposed to be breathing through it almost all the time. Your mouth is for eating, speaking, kissing, expression…. Not for breathing unless it's necessary.   If you are in the easy to nasal breathe category, then I have a basic program for you. Tape your lips shut. Yes, tape them shut. Typically, I recommend that you do this with medical tape such as the 3M micropore tape—either the paper or the plastic tape - whichever you prefer. They do make fancy lip tape that you can now search for online. It is designed for lip taping—but I still use the medical tape option. You can skip down below for the lip taping section.

Group No. 2 will be most people. If you can nasal breathe for one minute straight, you can get to the point of 90%+ with a little work. There are a variety of ways to improve and that is what this chapter is about.

Group No. 3 - No, not at all. There are two ways to go with this - first in about 95% of the time, nasal breathing can be obtained with functional exercises and nasal care techniques. For most, not using their nose for a long period of time - "nasal disuse" - results in the congestion of the tissue of the nose making it no longer possible to breathe through your nose by simply trying to do so. Therefore, I encourage you to work through this chapter, try all of it - and if at any time you find you CAN breathe through your nose calmly for one minute or more. Then keep with it until you can do so freely.

Five percent of the population will need some form of mechanical intervention to allow nasal breathing. This is typically due to severe deviated septums, excessive polyps, severely enlarged turbinates, extremely collapsed cartilage—physical blockages so severe that air simply cannot get through without intervention - again, 5% or less of these issues may require surgical intervention. But if you are one of them, DO IT and do it now! It is time to make that

ENT appointment and let them know that above all else, you need to breathe through your nose. This is NON-negotiable. And THEN, do everything you can to ensure you do not relapse. Relapse is common. You are not used to breathing correctly and you will continue to not do so unless you put in significant effort. Engage a myofunctional therapist (more described later) and Buteyko practitioner (ideally the same person) and let them help you. I cannot over emphasize how strongly I feel about this.

Answer these questions:

- While awake, do you mainly breathe through your nose or mouth?

- During the night, do you mainly breathe through your nose or mouth?

- Do you get chapped lips often?

- Do you wake up with a dry mouth?

- Do you often have bad breath?

- Do you keep water by your bed at night, need to drink a lot to stay hydrated?

- Do you clench or grind?

- Do you have persistent headaches?

The above questions will tell you if you should be paying closer attention to how you breathe and may not realize it. Chapped lips, a dry mouth, bad breath, clenching/ grinding your teeth, waking with headaches - these are signs of mouth breathing during the day or night.

I asked you which category you fell into for nasal breathing - did you guess, or do you know? Here is a good protocol for establishing nasal or mouth breather - the "Lip Seal Test".

This was presented in a paper titled *Assessment of Nasal Breathing Using Lip Taping: A Simple and Effective Screening Tool* in the International journal of Otorhinolaryngology; 2020 by Zaghi, Peterson, Shamtoob, et al. The basics are, using either lip tape, a tongue depressor, or holding a bit of water in your mouth —each will encourage the lip closed position, just hold it for three minutes and breathe through your nose. If you can sit calmly for those three minutes and breathe through your nose, you are in good shape for nasal breathing.

Your tongue should also be resting on the ROOF of your mouth. UP TOP. This is not a natural position for people. It will make your nasal breathing much easier and it is the proper resting place for your tongue. Just behind your front teeth on that little bump area ("the spot" for those familiar with that term) and then suctioned up the whole length of the palate. Proper breathing is lips closed, tongue up, teeth slightly together or slightly apart, breathing calmly and slowly through your nose. This is your goal. 90% or more of the time. Yes, you can do it. (Low tongue position promotes mouth breathing - and that is what we do not want!)

If you struggle with comfortable nasal breathing, I want you to do this Buteyko Breathing exercise to clear your nose. If you simply search the terms "nasal clearing Buteyko Breathing" online, you will come across videos showing you how to do this.

Here is the summary:

The following Exercise is very effective for decongesting your nose in just a few minutes:

1. Sit up straight.

2. Take a small breath in through your nose, if possible, and a small breath out. If your nose is quite blocked, take a tiny breath in through the corner of your mouth.

3. Pinch your nose with your fingers and hold your breath. Keep your mouth closed.

4. Gently nod your head or sway your body until you feel that you cannot hold your breath any longer.

5. Hold your nose until you feel a strong desire to breathe.

6. When you need to breathe in, let go of your nose and breathe gently through it, in and out, with your mouth closed.

7. Calm your breathing as soon as possible. Wait one minute or so and repeat for five or six times.

8. If someone can breathe through their nose for 1 minute, they can breathe through their nose all the time with proper exercises/training. If not, then true obstruction may exist.

Now that you know you CAN achieve nasal breathing, I will list some things you can do to improve upon this -make it easier, more frequent, more comfortable, more of a habit.... All the good things you need to succeed.

Lip Taping

I am putting this at the top of the list of things to do once you can establish the ability to nasal breathe because I have found it to be one of the best ways to ensure successful nasal breathing. You can do this during the day and at night. I typically have patients who are new to this start with short periods of time during the day to get used to it. As I mentioned in the first section, using simple medical tape such as 3M micropore (either paper or plastic) tape works well, though there is now special tape that you can find online fabricated for just this purpose. When using the micropore tape, I recommend beginning with a single vertical strip (tear a small piece that fits from just under your nose to just above your chin - then tear that in half long ways - you end up with a small strip to place vertically across your lips at the midline. You can find a half an hour sometime during the day to keep this in place and breathe only through your nose - when you are driving, working at your computer, reading, watching TV…. Really anything - and simply get used to that. You can graduate to taking the two thin vertical strips and making an "X" over your mouth for more stability. Once you are reasonably comfortable with this, it is time to move to night lip taping. Start with the small strips - for me using the "x" for more stability worked better and then I graduated to a full coverage of a whole strip horizontally across my mouth - and get the best sleep I have ever had as a result. The benefits from the first section should be enough to encourage you to start this practice as soon as possible. Another simple online search of the benefits of mouth/lip taping will get you tons of current information as well.

Nasal Valves

One common obstruction to comfortable nasal breathing is collapsed nasal valves. The nasal valve is at the entrance to your nose and is made of delicate cartilage that can become damaged and collapse, making it harder to get the air into the nostril. A test to determine if this might be your situation is called the "cottle maneuver". Place one or two fingertips on your cheeks on either side of your nose. Gently, press and pull outward. This temporarily opens the nasal valve. If doing this helps you inhale more easily through your nose, the nasal obstruction is likely to be in the nasal valve, in the front part of your nose.

If the cottle maneuver helped you breathe easier, something like the nasal strips that go across your nose or nasal cones will help improve your nasal breathing ability. During the typical day you are likely able to overcome the collapsed cartilage with minimal effort but at night, using the nasal strips or nasal cones will help open the passages. There are also now minor surgical techniques to restore the proper positioning of the cartilage. Whatever you decide, just make sure you are making it as easy and comfortable as possible to use that nose day and night.

Inflamed Turbinates & Allergies

50% of us have chronically inflamed turbinates. The turbinates are also called the nasal conchae. If the turbinates are too large, they can block airflow. This can be a temporary or a chronic condition. Some of the main causes are chronic sinus inflammation, environmental irritations, and seasonal allergies. Each of these conditions can cause the bone itself or the soft tissue of the turbinates to enlarge and swell. Whatever the cause, it is important to treat it.

Start with reducing allergens in the home - Here are some basic tips:

- Remove excess dust and pet dander from the home by vacuuming carpets, pillows, drapes, and furniture to remove dust.
- Keep pets out of your bedroom to reduce dander irritants.
- If you have fabric covered toys, 24 hours in the freezer can kill dust mites.
- A dust-proof cover over your mattress protects from dust-mites.
- No smoking. And definitely NOT indoors.
- Treat mold and mildew with specially formulated cleaners (think kitchens and bathrooms)
- Use a high efficiency particulate air (HEPA) filter indoors – especially in the bedroom where you sleep.

Additional Measures:

Sinus rinsing - this should be done ideally twice per day. The product I usually recommend is NeilMed Sinus rinse. They also have a netipot system that is quite good. Over the counter sinus sprays such as Ocean spray and Xlear are beneficial and safe to use.

There are medications that can be beneficial as well; remember you should check with your doctor to make sure there or no contraindications for your specific health issues. Medications to reduce seasonal allergies, such as Zyrtec, Claritin, or Allegra, oral decongestants, such as Sudafed (pseudoephedrine) can be helpful.

You may want to consider temporarily using medicated nasal spray decongestants to relieve nasal swelling. Flonase is a good option and available over the counter. However, these should not be used on a regular basis because they can cause bleeding and will be ineffective over time.

Allergies

If these at home measures are not adequately treating your allergies, it is time to see an allergist. Again, whatever you must do to be able to breathe through your nose you MUST do.

Nutrition

What we put into our bodies can do us harm and make us systemically inflamed which can result in poor breathing. Inflammation and oxidative stress are often the result of poor nutrition, toxins, and the environment. If we are eating and living in the modern world, we are systemically inflamed to some degree.

Following an anti-inflammatory diet will help many people significantly.

What is an anti-inflammatory diet?

According to a publication from Harvard medical school in 2020:

Inflammatory Foods

Try to avoid or limit these foods as much as possible:

- Refined carbohydrates, such as white bread and pastries

- French fries and other fried foods

- Soda and other sugar-sweetened beverages

- Red meat (burgers, steaks) and processed meat (hot dogs, sausage)

- Margarine, shortening, and lard.

Anti-Inflammatory Foods

An anti-inflammatory diet should include these foods;

- Tomatoes
- Olive oil
- Green leafy vegetables, such as spinach, kale, and collards
- Nuts like almonds and walnuts
- Fatty fish like salmon, mackerel, tuna, and sardines
- Fruits such as strawberries, blueberries, cherries, and oranges

To reduce levels of inflammation, aim for an overall healthy diet. If you are looking for an eating plan that closely follows the tenets of anti-inflammatory eating, consider the Mediterranean diet, which is high in fruits, vegetables, nuts, whole grains, fish, and healthy oils.

Myofunctional Therapy & Buteyko Breathing

What is a myofunctional therapist? A specialist trained to identify and correct abnormal oral-facial patterns by the way of practicing exercises to retrain the oral-facial complex to function properly while breathing, chewing, swallowing, and at rest. Just because you CAN breathe through your nose does not mean that you ARE. There are a variety of reasons for this and a myofunctional therapist can help identify them and get you on the right track. While there are many goals in myofunctional therapy, three of the most important ones are: nasal breathing, lips together, proper tongue position/function. Ideally, you can find someone who can provide myofunctional therapy as well as teach you Buteyko breathing techniques. The Buteyko breathing method focusses on the rhythm and rate of breathing, aiming to slow down the breathing rate and regulate the rhythm. A simple online search will result in a lot of information on this method and is worth the look.

Nasal Humming

Yes, this is humming through your nose and it has also shown benefits.... There is a study that shows a 15-fold increase in intranasal nitric oxide levels when performing nasal humming compared to a quiet exhalation - this study highlights a patient whose sinusitis was cured by nasal humming.... Might be the next big thing? There is a surprising amount of online information about this as well.

To Do:

Nasal Hygiene, twice per day

Use water, salt water, or xylitol sprays

Walk 10-15 minutes with lips closed, nasal breathing

Proper oral rest posture – tongue to the roof of the mouth & sealing the soft palate, lips together with slight pressure, teeth slightly apart or lightly touching, proper posture, and slow nasal breathing.

Over the counter treatments – start conservatively Nasal strips and nasal cones, nasal rinses and sprays.

How To Breathe

How to breathe? Isn't this something I just do all day and all night and do not have to think about it? Well for most, yes, but most are not doing it well - meaning it is happening in such a way as to promote illness and aging - when we can modify HOW we are doing it and promote health and longevity. Numerous ancient civilizations and religions have recognized and promoted the benefits of proper breathing. Once the modern world came about and there were ways that money could be made off products and pills - that's where attention, and funds, have been directed to. The art of breathing became overlooked and undervalued. It is time to take a fresh look and put it back at the top of the pyramid for health benefits value. Conscious breathing allows us to improve, maintain, and repair other unconsciously run systems of the body.

There are numerous techniques and methods that have been developed over the years. What has become obvious to me is that most focus on slow, long, deep breaths through the nose. I will briefly touch on the Buteyko method as I have found it very useful and am a practitioner of it. We will cover a few basic breathing exercises you can implement. In the ways to improve your nasal breathing section, the Buteyko nasal clearing exercise was introduced. I suggest doing this exercise multiple times a day until you are comfortable enough nasal breathing that you can implement the lip taping step. If you are not there yet, GO BACK. Being able to do this not optional.

A well-known researcher and scholar in this area was Konstantin Buteyko. He observed that a significant percentage of human beings are over breathing. It is so subtle, most of us do not know we are doing it. If we are over breathing, we are releasing too much carbon dioxide. If you remember your schooling, you will recall Bohr's affect which explains that a certain amount of carbon dioxide must be present for our red blood cells to release the bound oxygen into the tissues that need them. If we are over breathing and do not have adequate carbon dioxide in our tissues, the oxygen is not released as it should be. That is the basics. One of the significant ways to stop over breathing is to breathe through your nose. WITH YOUR MOUTH CLOSED. The air encounters greater resistance as it flows through your nasal passages and sinuses compared to breathing through your mouth. This automatically slows down our breathing and allows more carbon dioxide to be retained which enhances the release of oxygen. There are other huge benefits of breathing through your nose which we covered earlier.

What is considered medically normal today is anywhere between 12-20 breaths a minute, with an average intake of about half a liter per breath. For those on the high end of respiratory rates, that is about twice as much as it was. Most of us breathe too much and up to 1/4 of us are chronic over breathers. We have become conditioned with this unconscious habit.

The Buteyko method gets the body more comfortable with higher levels of CO_2, so that we will unconsciously breathe less during our resting hours and the next time we work out. As a result, we release more oxygen into our tissues, increase endurance, and better support all the functions in our bodies. If we aim to breathe as closely as possible to our metabolic needs, it almost always means taking in less air. It also means our heart rates & blood pressures improve, headaches disappear, those in good health feel better, and athletes see performance gains.

According to James Nestor, the Author of the best-seller *Breath*, the optimum amount of air we should take in at rest per minute is 5.5 liters. The optimum breathing rate is about 5.5 breaths per minute.   That is 5.5 second inhales and 5.5 second exhales. The perfect breath. Almost anyone, anywhere, can benefit from breathing this way for even a few minutes a day, much longer if possible: to inhale and exhale in a way that feeds our bodies just the right amount of air to perform at peak capacity.

One of the basic measurements of over breathing that the Buteyko method utilizes is called the Controlled Pause.

Note that in Buteyko Breathing, all breathing exercises and the Control Pause – which involves breath holding – are performed after an exhalation.

This information is taken directly from the Buteyko Clinic information, I am a fellow in Buteyko breathing and feel that sharing this information directly can vastly improve HOW you breathe.

To measure the extent of your relative breathing volume, a very simple breath hold test called the Control Pause (CP) is used.

For this you will need a watch or clock with a second hand.

1. Take a small silent breath in and a small silent breath out.

2. Hold your nose with your fingers to prevent air entering your lungs.

3. Count how many seconds until you feel the first signs of an air hunger.

4. Your inhalation at the end of the breath hold should be no greater than your breathing prior to taking the measurement.

5. Release your nose and breathe in through it.

If your breath in is disrupted, then you have held for too long and so have an inaccurate CP. Important thing to be aware of before we start:

1. The breath is taken after gently exhaling.

2. The breath is held until the first urges only. It is not a measurement of the maximum length of time that you can hold your breath.

3. The CP is a measurement of your breath hold time only. It is not an exercise to correct your breathing.

Remember that the CP is holding your breath only until the first urges. If you had to take a big breath at the end of the breath hold, then you held it for too long. The most accurate CP is taken first thing in the morning after waking up.

The lower your breath hold, the greater your breathing volume and the greater your anxiety symptoms. Big breathers are naturally more stressed than correct volume healthy breathers. A person with a high CP will be a lot more relaxed and calmer than a person with a lower

CP. People who experience panic or hyperventilation attacks are invariably big breathers. The objective is to reach a CP of 40 seconds.

Essential rules to make progress:

- You will feel better each time your CP increases by 5 seconds.

- If your CP does not change, you will not feel better. Your CP should increase by 3 – 4 seconds each week.

- The most accurate CP is taken first thing after waking. You cannot influence your breathing during sleep. As a result, this CP is the most accurate as it is based on your breathing volume as set by the respiratory center.

- Your CP as taken throughout the day will provide feedback of your symptoms at that time.

- Your goal is to have morning CP of 40 seconds for 6 months.

Three steps to increasing your CP:

STEP 1: Observe your breathing throughout the day and stop big breathing.

- Close Your Mouth

- Stop Sighing – swallow

- Apply gentle calm breathing

- Never hear your breathing during rest

STEP 2: Apply gentle reduced breathing

- Relaxation

- Stilling the mind

STEP 3: Take physical exercise with correct breathing (physical exercise is necessary to increase the CP from 20 to 40 seconds; more details further on).

STEP 1 is the foundation. Make the change to nasal breathing on a permanent basis, suppress your sighs, be aware of your breathing and ensure that it is quiet throughout the day. A regular sigh is enough to maintain chronic hyperventilation; therefore, it is very important to stop sighing by swallowing or holding your breath. Unless your foundation is strong, your progress will not be good. If you sigh and have taken a large breath, then hold your breath for ten seconds to counteract this. You will make progress by keeping your mouth closed but this will not be enough by itself. It is also necessary to reverse the over breathing habit that has developed over the years.

There is a TON more information on Buteyko breathing but this is where I want you to start. You can also get the booklet called *Close Your Mouth* by Patrick McKeown. A prior version called *Shut Your Mouth* has the same content. His book *The Oxygen Advantage* is a fantastic read on all the geeky science and how to improve your athletic performance using Buteyko methods.

Often, I will do breathing exercises that includes a slow and silent nasal breath in, a hold, then a slow and silent nasal exhale out, and another hold before the next slow and silent nasal intake. I recommend starting with the count of four seconds in, four second hold, four seconds out, four seconds hold and repeat for the duration of five minutes—set a timer if you need. Then move to five seconds and increase as you are comfortably able to do so up to the count of eight seconds in, eight second hold, eight seconds out, eight second hold. Twice per day, for five minutes. This is my method and is a form of a "box breathing" exercise. There are many exercises out there, I find this is the one that works best for me.

For the yoga practitioners out there, some yoga poses to aid in opening your rib cage and helping to achieve optimum breathing practices include camel pose, alternate nostril breathing, seated twists, triangle poses, three-part yogic breath, breath of fire, fish pose, and gentle back bends.

Fewer inhales and exhales in smaller volumes but carried deep into the lungs to promote diaphragmatic breathing is the key to improved health, endurance, and longevity. To breathe, but to breathe less.

You are now through the non-optional section of the book. Being able to breathe and do so properly is step ONE to improve your health, your sleep, your pain, and set you headed in the right direction. From this point on, I will be covering adjunct techniques and modalities that you can add in if you see fit for your specific needs. They are in no particular order.

The Importance of Sleep

—

There is so much about sleep that is important and so many factors that affect it. I am going to touch on a few basics only here. There is a lot of additional information out there and I encourage you to learn more.

There does not seem to be one major organ within the body, or process within the brain, that is not impaired when we do not get enough quality sleep.

We flip-flop between NREM and REM sleep throughout the night every 90-110 minutes. The ratio of NREM sleep to REM sleep within each cycle changes as the night/early morning progresses. In the first half of the night, most of our 90-minute cycles are consumed by deep NREM sleep and very little REM sleep. but as we transition through into the second half of the night, this seesaw balance shifts with most of the time dominated by REM sleep, with little, if any, deep NREM sleep.

A key function of deep NREM sleep, which predominates early in the night, is to do the work of weeding out and removing unnecessary neural connections. In contrast, the dreaming stage of REM sleep, which prevails later in the night, plays a role in strengthening those connections.

What a typical sleep cycle looks like:

- Stage one - lasts a few minutes, light, easy to wake from.

- Stage two - fairly light, brain waves begin to slow.

- Stage three & four - deeper sleep that is harder to wake from. Body grows and repairs and boosts immune function.

- REM - brain becomes active and dreams occur - brain is processing information and storing long term memories. This cycle repeats every 90-110 minutes; as sleep progresses through the night, REM cycles increase in length.

Some general guidelines:

- Sleep is the most important time for recovery. It replenishes physical and mental resources.

- Good sleep is a combination of enough sleep and quality of sleep.

- Good quality sleep includes–sleeping long enough, falling asleep in less than 30 minutes, waking up no more than once per night, and being awake for 20 mins or less after initially falling asleep.

Sleep Hygiene

—

What is sleep hygiene? One definition of hygiene reads "conditions or practices conductive to maintaining health and preventing disease". Here are things that you can implement to improve your sleep health and help prevent diseases that result from poor sleep quality &/or quantity.

Throughout the night, each of the stages of sleep provide the brain and body with different benefits. BOTH the quality AND the quantity of sleep are vitally important and there are active ways you can help to improve these. You may THINK you survive well off less than 7 hours of sleep but according to Matthew Walker (founder and director of the Center for Human Sleep Science at the University of California,

Berkeley) operating on short sleep — anything less than seven hours — impairs a host of brain and bodily functions. Once you get less than seven hours of sleep, you can measure marked impairments in both brain and body health. And those people who claim they can survive on six hours of sleep or less, unfortunately, are deluding themselves and their health. There are certain actions (or inactions) that you can put in place to help improve your sleep quality and quantity. These are the more common ones we recommend:

- Keep bedtime consistent - same time to bed and same time awake 7 nights a week. This may very well be THE most important thing you can do to improve your sleep.

- Set your thermostat at a max of 68. This is more important as you age or if you have insomnia.

- Use your bed ONLY for sleeping and sex.

- Create a bedtime routine.

- No caffeine after 12 noon

- Take breaks during the day. This lowers stress levels and allows your brain to slow down at the end of the day.

- Get at least an hour of sunlight every day.

- Exercise

- Do not take naps.

- Your bedroom furniture and décor should be calming.

- Blues and greens are calming.

- Cut out late night meals. If your body is busy digesting it is not resting.

- Cut alcohol at least 4 hours before bedtime.

- Cut smoking and other tobacco use.

- Raise the humidity in your room to help keep mucosal tissues from drying out. Consider an air purifier If you live in a noisy area, consider getting a white noise machine.

- Cut back on all screen time - including reading from a backlit device, computers, televisions, etc. at least one hour prior to bedtime.

- If you read prior to bed, try using an orange light in a reading lamp (white light suppresses melatonin release)

- Dim the lights one hour before bedtime. It sends your mind and body the signal that it is time to start winding down.

- Try warm herbal tea.

- Limit your use of sleeping aids or sleeping pills.

- Take a warm bath or shower prior to a cold bed.
- Leave your phone to charge in a different room. Meditate before bed. Sleep in total blackness (eye mask will work for this)
- Comfortable & hypoallergenic mattress, blankets, and pillow.
- Change your air filters every 3 months.
  - Lavender or chamomile scents

Wearables

—

Modern day technology offers some great methods to record and track a variety of metrics of our daily lives. With this knowledge comes power. The power to make changes in our behaviors to help improve our health metrics. Wearable technology that monitors our bodies on an ongoing basis can provide some very insightful data. These devices measure many things, I am considering sleep quality and quantity as one of the most important.

Features of these devices vary, but some common capabilities include:

- Sleep duration - by tracking the time you are inactive.

- Sleep quality - can detect interrupted sleep, tossing and turning.

- Sleep phases - some devices estimate phases based upon changes in metrics being monitored.

- Environmental factors - temperature, noise, light.

- Lifestyle factors - can enter information about exercise data, foods, stress levels.

In general, sleep trackers do not measure sleep directly (brain waves are not measured). Most sleep trackers measure sleep quantity and quality by using accelerometers - small motion detectors. The data is analyzed using an algorithm to estimate sleep time and quality. Heart rate and respiration - some sleep trackers estimate REM, deep, and light sleep stages by measuring heart rate (HR) and respiratory rate (RR). HR and RR vary widely during sleep, but they have a close relationship with each sleep stage. Respiration measurement can detect sleep disorders such as snoring and sleep apnea. Measuring heart rate variability (the difference in spacing between the beats - see section on this) - can also be detected - it is a measure of the autonomic nervous system activity.

When parasympathetic is dominant, heart rate (HR) is low and heart rate variability (HRV) is high. When sympathetic tone predominates, HR elevates and HRV generally declines from baseline. This is detected as a stressed state. The parasympathetic component of the ANS increases with sleep depth (stage 1 to stage 2 to stage 3) while the sympathetic component is related to awakening. REM sleep is characterized by variations in the sympathetic to parasympathetic tone balance. HRV can be used to measure physiological recovery during sleep.

I will list some of the common wearables people enjoy. I have tried all the following and compared them to high quality home sleep testing monitors. In general, the wearables give a good estimation of sleep quality. When you get into more details, such as sleep cycle specifics, the data is not as consistent. Overall, I would recommend any of the below devices for someone wanting to improve their sleep by becoming more aware of their nightly quality/ quantity. Small changes in behavior can result in significant improvements in sleep.

Circul by BodiMetrics (ring)

Water resistant

Calories

Pedometer

Sleep tracker

Heart rate monitor

Blood O2 Saturation

Battery life up to 12 hours

Used for wellness oximetry and blood oxygen night and day.
Overnight sleep tracking including SpO2%, HR, and 4 sleep stages (awake, light, deep, and REM)

Oura (ring)

Water resistant

Activity levels

Calories burned

Steps

Inactive times, naps

Resting Heart Rate

Heat Rate Variability
Body temp

Respiratory Rate

Light, Deep, REM sleep staging

Nighttime movement

Sleep timing and quality

Oura ring performed near-perfect for RHR (99.9) and extremely high for RHR (98.4) when compared to a medical grade ECG device. RR us accurate within 1 breath across the night. EMF safety - Bluetooth active less than 1% of the day and has an airplane mode available.

Whoop (wrist band)

Sleep stages

Sleep disturbances

Respiratory rate

Efficiency measures

Sleep duration & latency

Baseline and recovery sleep need - monitors trends and body recovery
Awake, light sleep, REM, Deep

HR & HRV

Measures "recovery" - using HRV

A recent study by U of A shows WHOOP offers a highly accurate commercially wearable for measuring sleep staging. - study shows highly accurate for RR, HR, and duration

Apple Watch

Blood oxygen sensor

HR & irregular rhythms

ECG app – sinus rhythm

Sleep - for best sleep tracking, you need to use outside apps. Below are some of my favorites.

- "Pillow" - uses a combination of movement, sounds, and HR to follow your patterns. Sleep stages focus (more than Autosleep) - deep, REM, light sleep, time in bed, time asleep. Delivers a sleep quality score. Tracks HR throughout night. Sleep algorithms are more detailed and sleep score/time asleep more in line with Fitbit.

- "AutoSleep" - works automatically - you do not have to tell it when you are getting in bed. Duration of sleep, a sleep rating, readiness score.
"readiness" - HRV and waking HR.
SPO2 throughout day and night.
Reports on sleep latency, awake/disrupted sleep, light sleep, still/restful, and deep sleep. Environmental Noise. Some reports show it might be a little more generous with sleep quality than "pillow" and fitbit. Better suited to those looking to get 8 hours a night and create good habits vs. getting into the science. "Sleep Bank" - keeps tabs on your week's sleep.

- "Sleep++" = popular om app store. Simple to use. Free. Data is bare bones. Very simple and data does not compare to other apps - data seems to show as a better night sleep than other apps - may be misleading – does show good long term trend data for duration and bedtime consistency.

- "Sleep Watch" - free. Tracks time, HR, and stages of sleep. Looks for dips in HR and correlates with restful sleep. HRV average - Sleep is ranked as disrupted, light, or restful (deep/REM combined?) and offers percentages. "sleep rhythm" - consistency of sleep times day to day. "% of restful sleep" vs time asleep - when body is most still. "heart rate dip" when sleeping. "sleep disruption" - based on activity sensed during sleep; can create "sleep reports" based on data gathered for 30 days. Fitness - VO2 max (amount of oxygen your body transfers to your blood - more it transfers, the healthier you are). Accelerometer and gyroscope to measure movement as well as HR during exercise; calories, standing, altimeter.

FIT BIT (watch/band)

Smart watch and tracker options

Heart Rate

Motion detector

Time asleep & sleep score

Deep, REM, light, awake sleep stages

Skin temperature

Estimated oxygen variation - looks for high variations that can indicate apnea.

The next few are some additional wearables that I do not have personal experience with, but some may find beneficial to investigate.

Garmin (watch/band)

Multiple styles with different focus

Activity tracking

Heart rate

Body energy monitoring

Pulse oximetry

Stress measurements

Respiratory rate

Sleep stages (deep, REM, light, awake)

Withings - this is not something you "wear" - it is a mat that you place under your mattress.

Wellue O2 (ring)

Blood oxygen saturation

Heart rate

Body motion

Vibrates when low O2 or abnormal HR detected.

Continuous tracking

Stand alone, no smart phone needed

LOOKEE (ring)

Oxygen saturation

Report for the whole night

Cheaper price point

Limited data

Amazon Halo (wrist band)

Home Stretches - TMJ

—

Rocabado's 6x6

Dr. Mariano Rocabado is a physical therapist and educator based out of Santiago, Chile. He is well known for his work with TMJ & craniofacial pain, bringing together dentists and physical therapists to enhance patient care.

These are his homecare exercises for patients suffering from TMJ, to help restore normal joint mobility in your jaw. These six exercises should be done with six repetitions each time, six times a day. (6 exercises x 6 repetitions x 6 times per day). Perform the exercises one after the other, it will take only a minute or two.

Exercise 1 - place your tongue on the roof of your mouth. Position the tip just behind your teeth and take six deep breaths.

Exercise 2 - keep your tongue on the roof of your mouth and open and close your mouth six times.

Exercise 3 - your tongue remains on the roof of your mouth and two fingers are placed on the chin to open your mouth against gentle resistance six times, then place your fingers on both sides of your jaw and open six times.

Exercise 4 - place your hands behind your neck and bend your chin down as if nodding your head.

Exercise 5 - Move your chin down and back, nodding as if making a double chin.

Exercise 6 - correct your posture by lifting your ribs and chest upward while squeezing your shoulder blades together.

Additional Home Stretches

These are some additional home care exercises we utilize. In general, if anything is causing pain, we do not want you to do it. I have patients repeat these exercises six times as well, three to six times per day. The exercises are designed to be done in order:

Tongue 'Clucking' – making a 'clucking' sound positions the tongue against the hard palate in the correct resting position for appropriate nasal and diaphragmatic breathing. Attempt to maintain appropriate tongue / jaw resting position throughout normal activity.

Controlled TMJ Rotation on Opening – Maintain tongue on the hard palate while opening and closing the jaw.
This position limits opening to rotational portions only and prevents excessive protrusion

of the mandible. This range of motion is to also be utilized during chewing, to control hypermobility.

Mandibular Rhythmic Stabilization – Apply resistance to opening, closing, and lateral deviation with the jaw in a resting position. The goal is to promote normal positioning of the jaw while maintaining appropriate postural alignment.

Controlled-Range of Motion (ROM) Lateral Deviation – From a resting jaw position, perform lateral deviation (slight side movement of the lower jaw) until the canine tooth on the lower jaw matches the canine tooth of the upper jaw. Palpate the condylar head (moving part of TMJ during this exercise) with 1 finger and the upper canine tooth with another finger to cue movement limitations, looking in a mirror may help.

Lateral Deviation + Functional Opening – From a resting jaw position, perform controlled-ROM lateral deviation followed by controlled- ROM opening. Movement may be monitored as above with self-palpation and positioning with a mirror.

Protrusion ROM – From a resting jaw position, perform protrusion (move jaw forward) of the mandible followed by retrusion (move jaw back) to a resting position, attempting to keep your jaw centered during motion. A mirror can help to perform the movement in midline and with good control.

Self-stretch into Opening – From a neutral posture and resting jaw position, open in midline and then provide a mild overpressure to the top and bottom teeth at end- range (pushing the teeth further apart, inducing a light stretch)

Nasal Breathing – Practice attaining and maintaining normal resting position of the jaw, with the tongue on the palate, lips closed, and teeth slightly apart.   This should be done at ALL times.

There are additional more advanced exercises that we may implement when indicated on a patient-by-patient basis, but everyone starts with the above (only if they can be performed with minimal to no pain)

Myofunctional Training

—

Contribution from Timbrey Lind,
RDH

It took me a while to get comfortable explaining to people what it is that I do because it is not a well-known field yet. The longer I practiced, the more I realized how easy it is to describe myofunctional therapy and how many people it can benefit. The main goals of Myofunctional therapy can be shrunken down to these three things: 1. Nasal breathing 2. Lips closed posture 3. Tongue up on the roof of the mouth.

Myofunctional therapy is the rehabilitation and re- training of the oral and facial muscles. This happens when our body has recruited other muscles to compensate for our primary muscle function. When this happens, our brain learns to stay in that pattern of using compensatory muscles instead of the correct and much stronger muscles that it should be using. Myofunctional therapy is a series of exercises you go through to not only activate but strengthen the primary muscles and get them working properly.

So, let us talk about why this is important. When we are not using the correct muscles to do simple functions such as swallowing and talking, we end up overworking the compensatory muscles and straining them. When this happens, it acts as a domino effect and puts unnecessary pressure elsewhere on our muscles and joints. Let us use an example to get a better visual. Let us say I see a patient with a tongue tie. That is when the skin underneath our tongue is too short and therefore, puts a natural strain on the normal use of the tongue. Some things the tongue should be able to do naturally (without fatiguing or moving your jaw) is clean your teeth, touch the roof of your mouth and all your molars with your mouth wide open, move your food side to side, lick all your teeth with your lips closed, and much more. When someone cannot do this, you probably have a short frenulum (skin underneath your tongue).

Some symptoms one might experience, if this is the case, is upper back and neck soreness, jaw pain, fatigue upon eating, headaches, digestive issues, gassiness, and the list can go on. This can ALL be caused from something as simple as a shortened frenulum, which is something we are born with. The thing is, if you are born with this, you do not know the difference of how it could feel, because you only know what you have. So, you experience the symptoms and cannot understand why this is all happening. If you are born with this, you go throughout your life compensating for all the movement your tongue may not be able to do naturally. Then those patterns are formed. This is where myofunctional therapy comes in and helps break those incorrect patterns and form new healthy ones for you and your body to function optimally. In this case specifically, the patient would go through a very simple and quick procedure to release that frenulum and give the tongue full freedom. After that, they would need to go through a series of exercises to help the tongue learn how to use this full-fledged freedom it was just granted after X number of years it was restrained. The tongue and facial muscles would need to re-learn how to do all the simple functions such as swallowing, talking, resting, etc.

Some main symptoms of a myofunctional disorder range anywhere from jaw joint pain, speech impediments, stomach aches from an incorrect swallow, insomnia, snoring, chronic mouth breathing, headaches, neck pain, and thumb sucking.

A huge part of myofunctional therapy is also teaching nasal breathing. Most of the time, when we suffer from weak oral and facial muscles, we end up breathing mainly through our mouths. When this happens, it creates a domino effect of a lot of negative symptoms that can have a major effect on your facial development and immunity and even anxiety, to name a few.

Through using myofunctional therapy, you learn proper tongue posture which encourages nasal breathing. This is a much healthier alternative to mouth breathing for a copious number of reasons.

Heartrate Variability

—

What is heart rate variability (HRV)? You
know how your heart rate might be 60 beats
per minute or 80 beats per minute? That is the
average. HRV is literally the variation between
your heart beats. It is measured in milliseconds.
Meaning one beat might occur a few
milliseconds before the next. In general, the
greater the variability between beats, the
greater your ability to respond to stress and the
fitter you are. It is a measurement of your
autonomic nervous system.

Your autonomic nervous system is composed of
two branches. The parasympathetic (rest, digest,
and recovery) and your sympathetic
(fight/flight) branches. The parasympathetic
system elicits slower heart rates, slower
breathing, a more relaxed state. The sympathetic

system is activated during stress and exercise, increasing your heart rate and breathing. Heart rate variability is affected by these two branches constantly sending signals to your heart. When you have a high heart rate variability it means your body is sensitive to both inputs. You can adapt and perform for what is required of you.

In today's constant stress promoting lifestyles, it is typical that the sympathetic nervous system is over activated and is dominant most of the time. It sends out stronger signals. When we need to run from a predator this is a good thing, it is also a good thing when you are running a marathon and need these resources directed properly. However, we often see an overactive sympathetic nervous system because of day-to-day non-threatening events (traffic on the way to work? Angry coworker? Overdue bill? Too much work and too little time? Not enough work? COVID worries?).

The list goes on and on… and our system gets stuck in what can be called sympathetic overdrive. We get used to living this way. The problem is our body is working hard all the time leaving fewer resources available to dedicate to rest and repair - we literally cannot get into a physiological place where our body can do what it is designed to do - heal itself.

I bet you want to know what a healthy HRV is. I cannot tell you. It is extremely individualized. What is more important is your individual variation. If you measure your HRV for a period of time, you will see a range that is typical for you. When you are lower in that range, you are most likely in a more stressed state (or at least your body is even if you do not feel it) and when you are higher in that range, it can indicate that your system has the resources available it needs to function at its optimum.

Athletes often use HRV to determine their workouts - if they are in the lower HRV range, then they need to take it easy because their body needs extra help to be its best. If their HRV is higher than average, they can push it and rely on their body to respond well to the increased training.

So, what does this mean for you? This is not just about fitness. It is about your body being able to dedicate its resources to help you be healthier, combat pain, combat illness, improve your sleep…. It is a way you can help set your body up to help you achieve your goals. You can measure this, and you can affect it by the choices you make. It is not pre-determined.

There are many factors in our lives that affect our HRV. Biological factors you do not have control over such as your age (generally HRV declines with age), gender (men typically have higher HRV's), genetics, and any health conditions you may suffer from. The good news is that your lifestyle choices also have a big impact, factors such as diet/nutrition, alcohol consumption, sleep habits, and stress.

There are gobs of information on improving your HRV for athletes. All it takes is a simple google search and you will find recommendations such as pay attention to your training and give your body time to recover, stay hydrated, avoid alcohol, eat a healthy diet, get quality sleep, stick to a schedule. By the way, that advise is excellent advice for everyone - not just the athletes. There are additional ways you can improve your HRV. If it is typically the sympathetic branch of the autonomic nervous system that is overactive, then it makes sense to consciously try to activate the parasympathetic branch. You can do this through diaphragmatic breathing - even as little as one minute a few times a day has been shown to be a benefit. One of the easiest, and one of my favorite ways to improve your breathing and activate the parasympathetic system is covered in the "how to breathe properly" section.

If you are someone who likes to see the data and see your improvements, the best source I have come across both for information as well as for technology to help you track is through the company "HeartMath". They focus on what they call "the heart-brain communication". Research has shown that the heart communicates to the brain in four major ways: neurologically (through the transmission of nerve impulses), biochemically (via hormones and neurotransmitters), biophysically (through pressure waves) and energetically (through electromagnetic field interactions). The neural communication pathways interacting between the heart and the brain are responsible for the generation of HRV. You can literally train your body to alter its HRV by using thoughts and breathing. I highly encourage you to check out www.heartmath.com. There is literature, training, products and more. It is one more aspect, and an important aspect we are finding, how you can help yourself. The first step in most of the techniques developed by the HeartMath Institute is called Heart- Focused Breathing, which includes placing one's attention in the center of the chest (the area of the heart) and imagining the breath is flowing in and out of the chest area while breathing a little slower and deeper than usual. With conscious control over breathing, an individual can slow the rate and increase the depth of the breathing rhythm. They have technology that can help you track your progress in improving your HRV.

Nutrition & Supplements

—

Inflammation, Lifestyle, & Nutrition

Inflammation can be either acute or chronic. Acute inflammation is how our body heals itself and is necessary for our survival. It is how we fight infections and heal ourselves. Signs of it include swelling, warmth, redness, pain in the tissues/joints in response to an injury. Chronic inflammation happens when our immune system prolongs the process. Your immune system thinks the body is under constant attack, so it keeps fighting. Chronic inflammation is associated with many long-term health problems such as heart disease, cancer, bowel diseases, diabetes, and arthritis.

Chronic systemic inflammation can be a large contributor to chronic pain and sleep issues. It is something that we have some degree of control over, mainly by adjusting our nutrition, exercise, and possibly supplements.

Living in today's world, all of us, to some degree, are "inflamed". Pollutants, allergies, toxins, the food we eat, the water we drink, among other every day experiences are some of the contributors. It often goes unnoticed and can affect our overall health drastically. So how do you know if you have chronic inflammation? There are blood tests which measures a protein that is elevated with inflammation (CRP = C reactive protein). There are other methods to measure as well, but this is the most common way.

Diet and exercise have a huge impact on managing chronic inflammation. A healthy diet and exercise also help maintain healthy weight and improve your sleep - both in turn help curb inflammation as well. You have probably heard of "anti-inflammatory diets". Certain foods are associated with promoting inflammation in your body. The most obvious of these foods include simple sugars (think soda, candy, fruit juices, sports drinks). Other foods in this category include refined carbohydrates (think white bread, pasta) and processed meats. Anti-inflammatory foods (foods that can lower inflammation) include foods high in antioxidants (berries, cherries, plums, red grapes, turmeric, green tea, and dark green leafy vegetables). These are just some examples of how you can alter your nutrition to help fight systemic inflammation. As for exercise, studies have shown that just twenty minutes of moderate intensity exercise can have an anti-inflammatory effect.

According to the Mayo Clinic, here are some simple rules of thumb for anti-inflammatory eating:

- Eat more plants. Whole plant foods have the anti- inflammatory nutrients that your body needs. So, eating a rainbow of fruits, veggies, whole grains, and legumes is the best place to start.

- Focus on antioxidants. They help prevent, delay, or repair some types of cell and tissue damage. They are found in colorful fruits and veggies like berries, leafy greens, beets, and avocados, as well as beans and lentils, whole grains, ginger, turmeric, and green tea.

- Get your Omega-3s. Omega-3 fatty acids play a role in regulating your body's inflammatory process and could help regulate pain related to inflammation. Find these healthy fats in fish like salmon, tuna, and mackerel, as well as smaller amounts in walnuts, pecans, ground flaxseed and soy.

- Eat less red meat. Red meat can be proinflammatory. Are you a burger lover? Aim for a realistic goal. Try substituting your lunchtime beef with fish, nuts, or soy-based protein a few times a week.

- Cut the processed stuff. Sugary cereals and drinks, deep-fried food, and pastries are all pro-inflammatory offenders. They can contain plenty of unhealthy fats that are linked to inflammation. But eating whole fruits,

- veggies, grains, and beans can be quick if you prep ahead for multiple meals.

Blood Work

——

We are all familiar with getting our blood drawn to help evaluate our health. Beyond the basic traditional blood work, there are additional tests that provide much more individualized and valuable information to help you not only "get well" but also allow prevention (the best medicine).

The blood test that I currently like the most is through "SpectraCell Laboratories". Their micronutrient test measures 31 specific micronutrients - vitamins, minerals, amino acids, antioxidants, and metabolites - our bodies use these to perform every biological function. Regardless of the cause, this test will uncover micronutrient deficiencies. Decisions can then be made to encourage prevention by correcting these deficiencies. There can often be no clinical symptoms associated with deficiencies until over time the progression can lead to much larger health problems. I am a big proponent of knowing what your current micronutrient levels are and addressing any deficiencies.

Many of the commonly accepted causes of disease (inflammation, genetics, gut issues) are manifestations of micronutrient deficiencies. Some examples include inflammation, poor gut health, low immunity, hormonal imbalance, increased susceptibility to environmental toxins, and non-restorative sleep.

What truly makes SpectraCell's version of testing unique is that it measures the functional level and capability of micronutrients within the white blood cells. Other tests measure the presence of nutrients outside of the cells, within the serum of the blood. Splicing the white blood cells and evaluating the internal makeup of the micronutrients gives a longer-term assessment that looks at the actual performance of the micronutrients. It does not matter if they are simply floating around in the blood if they are not doing the work they need to be doing inside of your cells.

Getting this information is one thing. You will want to talk with someone who is well educated in analyzing the results. Many factors come into play when considering adding supplementation. If you are interested in obtaining this test, we can help guide you to the proper resources we believe to be among the best.

Vitamins & Sleep

—

Dr. Stacia Gominak is a neurologist who focuses on sleep. She has found there is a vital connection between sleep and healing. She has also found that optimum vitamin D levels produce better sleep, no matter what the sleep levels. Most of us in modern day society are deficient in vitamin D. Which is not a vitamin, but a hormone that is made when UVB light interacts with our skin. Dr. Gominak also states that a longstanding vitamin D deficiency typically means you will have a vitamin B deficiency too. This is because your gut bacteria are affected and damage to your microbiome means that the B vitamins are not produced properly. B vitamins also affect our sleep, and a deficiency will fuel the cycle of poor sleep and more. She goes on to state that you must heal your B's - when your gut bacteria are weak, you will feel bad.

Dr. Gominak has developed a program called "Right Sleep" and has helped many people get better quality and quantity of sleep. Her program involves determining where you are starting from and creating a program of customized supplementation of B's and D vitamins.

After your gut bacteria are restored to health and properly producing their B vitamins, all you will need to sustain is proper levels of vitamin D (whether producing it naturally or with supplements added in). I have seen success with helping patients manage their pain (you can't heal if you don't get that proper sleep) and their sleep issues. It's another tool we have access to, and I suggest you do a simple google search of Dr. Gominak and her "Right Sleep" program.

CBD, THC &
Phytocannabinoids

—

Note that this section has been written for general information only and you should consult with your medical professional for your specific needs/concerns.

I am a big believer in using CBD and related cannabinoids. This topic deserves more explanation as it is unknown or confusing to many people.

To start with, we all have a system of receptors throughout our body that respond to these compounds. It is our endocannabinoid system. When we refer to "endocanabinoid", these are compounds we make within our body and our body has receptors designed to interact with them. This was unknown until relatively recently and since that time, we have been learning and researching quite a bit. The information I am giving you here is to the best of my knowledge to date and likely will become more involved and improved over time.

CBD vs THC

The Cannabis species of plant includes both the marijuana and hemp plants. THC comes from Marijuana and CBD comes from Hemp. They are both compounds called "phytocannabinoids" (cannabinoids that come from plants). It was found that these phytocannabinoids can also react with our endocannabinoid (within our body) receptors. The research and use of phytocannabinoids have been banned until recently.

Not all phytocannabinoids are the same. There are over 100 already identified (these compounds from plants that interact with our receptors). All phytocannabinoids, including CBD and THC, produce effects in the body by interacting with the receptors. THC is psychoactive & produces a "high". CBD is completely non-psychoactive and is known for its health benefits. When combined with THC, it can suppress and numb down some of the mind-altering qualities of THC. Pure CBD products, by law, must contain .03% or less of THC. Different % combinations can produce different effects for people.

In my office, I only work with CBD & CBG & other non-psychoactive products though I do believe for some patients adding in THC can be beneficial - but this is outside of my scope of clinical recommendations.

CBD is not just another supplement. Cannabidiol (CBD) is one of over 100 compounds found in hemp and marijuana. It is non-psychoactive. This is the part of the plant that gets you healthy, not high. CBD is extracted as an oil from cannabis. Research has been suggesting that it can help alleviate several medical issues in a lasting and effective manner. A question to ask is what do we all consider "health"? Is it just the absence of disease? Or is it that all our bodily systems are functioning to the best of their abilities which means that they can return to proper balance on their own, when they are disturbed or knocked out of balance. This is the body being able to maintain homeostasis.

Having resiliency to bounce back.

What is the ECS?

The Endocannabinoid System (ECS) is perhaps the most important physiological system involved in establishing and maintaining human health. I never learned about the ECS in school. I learned about all the other body systems but the one system that oversees all of these other systems wasn't discovered until the 1990's in Israel.

It was named after the plant (cannabis) that led to its discovery (they were researching how THC affects the body) and this led to the ban of the whole plant and all the compounds within it (a discussion for another time). The Endocannabinoid system's function is massive. Endocannabinoids are some of the most versatile and widespread molecules. In fact, there are more receptors involved in the ECS than all other receptors in our body combined. The system plays a major role in balancing many important functions; maintaining homeostasis appears to be its primary function. The ECS exists in any animal with a vertebra, including fish, reptiles, birds, and mammals. The role of the ECS is to bring balance to our tissues, including the heart, digestive, endocrine, immune, nervous, and reproductive systems. It is vital to maintain health and wellness. This is our body's main way of providing that resiliency against systems out of balance and returning us to overall physical homeostasis or overall health.

The Basic Components of the ECS

The basic components, very simplified, of the ECS are Endocannabinoids (ligands/binding molecules), receptors, and Enzymes. Endocannabinoids are produced naturally within the body (endo = within) and they bind with the cannabinoid receptors, located on cell membranes, to induce actions within the cell needed to carry out essential life functions. As soon as the body is thrown out of balance, it signals the endocannabinoids and cannabinoid receptors for assistance. There are two main receptors in our body, known as CB1 and CB2. CB1 is found mainly in the brain and nervous system, and in peripheral tissues and organs. CB2 is a peripheral receptor mainly the immune system.

Our Endocannabinoids

There are two main endocannabinoids that we produce. They are produced when and where they are needed, serving as messengers to act on neurons throughout the body.

AEA (Anandamide) is known as the bliss molecule. This was the first endocannabinoid discovered by researchers. It impacts every system. It is a partial agonist of both CB1 & CB2. It is broken down by FAAH enzyme and has a short half-life (less than 5 min). It functions in a vast array. Sleep deprivation results in AEA deficiency and results in memory issues the next day.

Less is known about 2-AG (2arachidonoylglycerol). It was identified a few years after AEA. It is a full agonist of both receptors & the primary ligand for the CB2 receptors. It is metabolized by the enzyme MAGL. It is focused in the gut and neuronal system. Levels of 2-AG can be affected by an unhealthy gut.

Our Receptors

Once manufactured, endocannabinoids attach to receptors. Receptors are located throughout the body. There are more cannabinoid receptors present in the body than all the other neurotransmitter receptors put together. When they are activated, it can be by our internally made endocannabinoids, as well as by the phytocannabinoids found in hemp and cannabis.

The CB1 receptor is concentrated in the brain and central NS but also is found in other parts of our bodies. They deal with thinking, mood, appetite, memories, pain, emotion, movement, coordination, and many other functions. The CB2 receptor is mostly in the peripheral organs especially cells associated with the immune system & gut. They affect inflammation and pain.

When our ECS is Deficient

The links between a deficiency in the functioning of the ECS and numerous medical disorders have been quite surprising. Researchers believe that the underlying cause of many ailments, particularly those related to the immune system and inflammation, could be a disorder referred to as clinical endocannabinoid deficiency. The theory of clinical endocannabinoid deficiency suggests that in some cases the body does not produce enough endocannabinoids or enough receptors, or there is too much of the breakdown enzymes. As a result, the ECS does not function properly and the body becomes unbalanced, allowing diseases & symptoms to arise. Dr. Ethan Russon first proposed this in 2004 - suggested that this could explain why supplementing Phytocannabinoids found in plants like hemp were proving effective at alleviating some conditions. It is suggested that ECS deficiency could be so common and prevalent that it could be the explanation for several medical conditions that are not fully understood nor have a cure.

The Entourage Effect

The Entourage Effect describes how using more than one part of the plant has shown to have greater benefits. You get the benefit from the individual components PLUS added benefits that you would not get unless you use them both. For example, while CBG is a direct activator of the CB2 receptor, CBD will then actually adjust the resulting changes to the physiology- it can dial it up or dial it down, but it needs the CBG to activate the receptor. "Full Spectrum" refers to using "all of the plant" and will give you the most benefits. Products can be created with different percentages of different phytocannabinoids and other components of the plant which results in different benefits.

How CBD Works

Unlike most active ingredients which only adjust in one direction, either lowering an element or raising it, CBD is more of a buffer and acts multidirectional - this is part of what makes it so unique. Therefore, when the body cannot maintain homeostasis, CBD can act in many ways to assist. It allows our Endogenous

Cannabinoid System (ECS) to work properly and self-regulate when it is not able to on its own.

Anyone in today's modern world has a system that is inflamed to some degree - be it chronic stress, chronic infections, environmental toxins, pharmaceutical use, unhealthy lifestyle, non-nutritious food, etc. - these have all shown to have a large effect on our physiology and the ECS is no exception.

CBD can correct imbalances by either enhancing or inhibiting how a receptor transmits a signal by working at the level of the individual cells. This is very different than pharmaceuticals. Pharmaceuticals work at the level of the symptoms you are having. With CBD, we are treating the causes of imbalance by allowing the body to help itself vs. chasing the symptoms with pharmaceuticals.

CBD is indirectly responsible for better sleep mostly because it stops inflammation on the cellular level.

Research has shown CBD's effect on sleep:

- CBD may help reduce anxiety, which is a major cause of insomnia.

- CBD induces alertness, but also appears to help increase overall sleep time at night.

- CBD helps with sleep onset in pain patients CBD may help reduce insomnia.

- CBD's alertness promoting property is powerful enough to counteract the sedative properties of the same dose of THC.

- CBD may help improve REM Sleep Disorder.

CBD & Pain Management

In the management of pain, studies have shown that CBD not only serves as an anti-inflammatory agent, but also encourages the pathways of the ECS to better facilitate its "messages" in the form of proteins and enzymes. CBD has been observed to assist cells in their regeneration processes. It can be used to reduce inflammation at the site of injury (a sprained ankle, for example), or for chronic pain caused by pinched, irritated, or injured nerves (called neuropathy). Several studies show that CBD can effectively decrease the prescribed dose of opioids for pain management. CBD can also lessen the symptoms of withdrawal from opioids.

CBD & Inflammation

Inflammation is a bodily response to harmful stimuli. Many things can cause this response in your body, which is why inflammation is more a "warning sign" rather than a disease itself. It typically correlates with many different diseases in humans.

Inflammation is a generic response to a threat to your health. Your body activates your immune system as you try to fight off the "attacker." Unfortunately for most people, their habits or modern living are what causes the inflammation in the first place. CBD and its fellow cannabinoids target certain cytokines – such as the pro- inflammatory ones – and silences them. It can take the very cause of the inflammation signal and simply tell it to quiet down.

Ongoing research is showing that cannabinoids have an adaptive, immunomodulating effect. This means that rather than just suppressing immune activity, they can bring an over- or under-reacting immune system back into balance. This means it may play an integral role in managing autoimmune diseases. There is a lot of research in this area currently. Wouldn't it be great if we could calm down our "modern living" inflammation response? Using effective natural therapies first, then work to identify the causes of our personal inflammation and get rid of them, whether they are stress related, nutrition-relation, or due to exposure to environmental toxins. And we can even be less anxious about all of it because CBD enhances GABA's natural calming effects as well!

CBD & Dosing

Phytocannabinoid compounds need to be SELF-titrated to find the correct dosage for each patient. Everyone's endocannabinoid system is different. Some people's endocannabinoid system is very sensitive & reacts to low doses. Some have a very tolerant endocannabinoid system and will react to only high doses. Yet other people's endocannabinoid system may vary with the time of the day or the time of the month. Always start at a low dose and titrate up slowly. Stop when you arrive at the dose that works for you and continue at that dose.

Products

It is truly the wild west out there with regards to different phytocannabinoid products. They are currently unregulated by the FDA; therefore, you need to be cognizant that products might not be or do what they claim. Either become more knowledgeable yourself or work with someone you trust who does understand how it all works. In general, you can find products as edibles, tinctures, topicals, and smokables. Some important things to look for in the products include the hemp being grown organically on USDA certified soil and US Hemp Authority certified, that the product is water soluble, a full spectrum hemp oil, processed using high pressure Carbon Dioxide (CO_2), and having a certificate of authenticity (COA). Third party monitoring is a very important quality control process. This means that an outside company tests and certifies the contents of the product. Typically, you can find a bar code or way to look up the product and see what exactly is in what you are purchasing.

Epigenetics

You likely have heard the term "epigenetics". Epigenetics refers to the ability to control changes in our gene function without a change to our DNA. It's how we can influence our health in spite of whatever our DNA encodes for us. It is a myth that genes create disease, and you are determined to end up a certain way. This is what science used to say but now we know that our environment (including choices we make), by activating or deactivating particular genes, is the most causative factor in producing disease. 95% of all illnesses are related to lifestyle choices, chronic stress, and toxic factors in the environment. There are several studies on identical twins (exact same gene sequence) who have had very different experiences when it comes to their health and longevity.

The external environment therefore influences our internal environment. In addition, by changing our internal state of being, we can overcome the effects of a stressful or toxic environment so that certain genes do not become activated. We may not always be able to control all the conditions of our external environment, but we have a choice in controlling our internal environment. Epigenetics means that we can signal our genes to navigate our future. The latest research shows that different genes are activated at different times - they are always in flux and being influenced. In reality, genes don't get turned on and off. They are activated by chemical signals and they express themselves by making various proteins which have affects throughout the body.

Just by changing our thoughts, feelings, emotional reactions, and behaviors (for example, making healthier lifestyle choices with regard to nutrition, stress level, exercise, etc.), we send our cells new signals, and they make different proteins. If we stay in the same toxic state of anger, in the same situations that cause depression, in the same hyper stressed state of anxiety, or in many of the other unhealthy states that modern living offers up - those redundant chemical signals keep pushing the same genetic results and ultimately this causes certain diseases.

But what if the situation or environment is not changing? Good news! We can signal the body emotionally and begin to alter a change in genetic events. Through thought and emotion alone, we can make changes - studies have shown that emotions can turn on some gene sequences and turn off others. When you experience an event in your mind, mentally rehearsing it, you can feel the emotions without an actual event. The circuitry in your brain changes and you can change how your genes are activated and respond which means you can change your body and how your future unfolds. Seems far-fetched, especially when you are "stuck", but it is true!

Let us talk about the autonomic nervous system again. We do not have to consciously think about breathing, our body temperature, our heart beating, our digestive system breaking down the nutrients we consume… our body does this all on its own. Millions of processes within our body that we do not think about and our system does them on its own. What about our emotional responses? Do we let our body just take control? That can be a disastrous choice and it is a choice we actually have. We develop conditioned responses over time (think about Pavolv and his dogs). Our emotions and responses occur automatically; our body responds with little or no conscious effort. What happens if we begin to anticipate some unwanted future event or obsess about a worse- case scenario? We are pre-programming our body to experience the event that has not even happened. The body does not know the difference between the actual event and our just thinking about it. Most of us are either thinking ahead, or reliving the past, in our current thoughts. If we are focused on an unwanted past or dreaded future event that means we are living in a stress and survival mode. This can become an addictive mindset that causes our adrenal glands to release high amounts of stress hormones resulting in an unhealthy chemical imbalance we are not designed to chronically experience. Whether we are running from a lion, stressing over traffic, bumping into an ex, remembering a past event, or anticipating a future one - we produce the same physiological stress response.

This kind of repetitive stress is harmful. We are not designed to have our stress response turned on with such frequency and for long durations. When we turn on the stress response, and we cannot turn it off, we are headed for some sort of breakdown in our body. Our immune system cannot keep up and growth and repair do not happen as they should.

Overproduction of stress hormone creates emotions of anxiety, depression, anger, fear, and similar negative emotions. The more we live engulfed in stress hormones, the more it becomes addictive - we can literally get addicted to being in a stressed state, it gives us a chemical boost and rush of energy. We can find it hard to change this. This can literally lead to our thoughts making us physically sick.

If our thoughts can make us sick, they can also make us well. If we can un-memorize the negative emotions causing the stress, we can stop signaling the genes in this manner. We can consciously signal them in a way that promotes healing and health.

Meditation & Breathwork

—

As we discussed earlier, by controlling our breathing, we can give power back to the parasympathetic branch of our autonomic nervous system. This involves taking this long, slow breaths through the nose activating the vagus nerve and diaphragmatic breathing.

Meditation is a great way to accomplish this as well. Most of the pain and sleep deprived patients I treat roll their eyes (at least internally) when I bring this up. They have "tried it" and "it didn't work". I am suggesting you try it again, maybe take a different approach. You do not have to sit there and clear your mind, focusing on breathing slowly in and out of your nose - but if this works for you then by all means, do it! What has worked for me, and countless others, is using tools and techniques to help calm the mind. I say "calm" not "clear" because having thoughts is just fine and is most likely going to happen. There are apps out there that I especially find beneficial, and they have a variety of ways to approach this. My favorite apps as of this writing include "calm", "breethe", "sounds true", "headspace", and "mindfulness". There is free content as well as a wider variety of paid content for most of these. I also have enjoyed "Deepak and Orpah's" app which includes a variety of extended day meditation options. I find using the "guided" meditations gives me something to focus on.

Another way I have found to tap into the parasympathetic system and calm my mind is using the products from "heartmath". They have an inexpensive product that connects to your iPhone or laptop and can give you feedback which literally can train your body and mind to relax upon command. This is an extremely useful tool. It is a version of biofeedback technology.

According to medical news today, biofeedback therapy is a non-drug treatment in which patients learn to control bodily processes that are normally involuntary, such as muscle tension, blood pressure, or heart rate. There is even a version whereas you gain more control over these bodily processes, you can view a black and white drawing slowly turn to color. I think this is a great way to dip your toe into this if you are one of the meditation eye rolling types. More and more research is coming out about how helpful meditation and breath work are to overall health and longevity.

Red Light Therapy

——

*Contribution from Timbrey Lind,
RDH*

Red light therapy is a way to biochemically strengthen your cells, which includes your mitochondria. And again, the mitochondria are the powerhouse of the cell, where all the energy is created. When we can increase the function of the mitochondria, with red light therapy, then the cell has more energy per say, to do its job which is to create energy. When a cell has energy, it can put it towards healing and regeneration. Other benefits include reducing inflammation, stimulates healing of wounds, aids in relief and pain of arthritis, helps decrease skin issues such as psoriasis, builds collagen and helps break down scar tissue.

If you decide to get a red light, there are a few things to know. A red-light range is visible light of 600-670 nm range (works superficially on skin). Superficial red-light therapy will contribute to improved skin complexion and enhanced wound healing.

Then there is near infrared, which is nonvisible in 800-880 nm range (works deeper on a cellular level). This is a more effective way with multiple benefits such as athletic performance and recovery, eye health, reduces inflammation and oxidative stress, improves mitochondrial function and energy, to name a few. Near infrared light also stimulates cytochrome c oxidase enzymes in the mitochondria which increases nitric oxide production.

If you want to look up studies on red light therapy, they use the term "photobiomodulin" is the term used in the literature reporting health benefits.

EMF Exposure

—

Contribution from Timbrey Lind, RDH

With the world relying on so much technology in this day and age, we are being overexposed with EMF's. EMF is an acronym that translates to Electromagnetic Field that is produced by moving electric charges. To give you an example and comparison, since the beginning of the Universe, the sun has sent out waves that create electric and magnetic fields, or radiation. This is something we can see, its visible light. After scientists studied this, they mimicked in with other power lines, cell phone towers, televisions, microwaves, wi-fi routers, computers, Bluetooth devices, and cell phones. These are not EMF exposures we can see, like the light of the sun, but more so something our body can feel and responds to, mostly in a negative way. Our body is made of electrons and therefore, reacts to electrical fields.

Scientists have stated that they are not concerned with this exposure yet the World Health Organization's International Agency for Research on Cancer (IARC) states that after conducting some studies, EMF's are "possibly carcinogenic to humans". The IARC believes that some studies show a possible link between EMF's and cancer in people.

Some ways your body would be telling you that you are being overexposed is:

- Sleep disturbances
- Lack of concentration
- Restlessness and anxiety
- Skin burning, tingling, or itching
- Headaches
- Depression
- Tired/fatigued

Again, because our society relies so much on technology nowadays, a lot of the exposure we come across is not within our control. So, I am going to give you some ideas that will help you control your environment better to help protect you and lower your EMF exposure.

Check how many cell towers are around you (antennasearch.com). This is a great thing to do to get an idea of how much exposure is around you.

Purchase a basic EMF meter to find out the exposure within your home. The most efficient one I have found that does not break the bank is by Safe Living Technologies called the Cornet ED88TPlus on amazon. Its $190, but a great investment as you will use it often and anywhere. Go around your house and find the "hotspots". This will usually be around a wifi router, microwave, etc.

After you have found where the most exposure is coming from, reduce it by:

- Turning off your wifi when you do not need to use it.

- Put your phone in airplane mode when you do not need to use it.

- Simply distancing yourself from the major EMF exposures will help reduce exposure.

- Sleeping with your phone in another room

- Not carrying your phone anywhere on your body

There have been several products developed to help "block" the EMF's and/ or change the electric field so that it is not negatively affecting you. These companies are Soma Vedic and Qu Wave.

They have created EMF blocking cases for certain products.

Grounding every day, multiple times a day. I will go into depth about this later, but what this means is coming in contact with the earth's surface. Skin to earth.

Using a body voltage meter will be able to show you the effects EMF's have on the body. You will also be able to see if grounding is working for you. Gen El Body voltage meter for $120 is a great one I've found.

Something to keep in mind if you live in a city, there tends to be a lot of "dirty electricity" and therefore grounding can make it worse for you. For dirty electricity, having filters can help a bit (Greenwave dirty electricity filters $30). They also offer a meter that helps you find out if/ where you have dirty electricity.

These ideas are a great start to reducing your EMF exposure and getting you feeling better and living a longer, healthier life. Even if you are not a believer in EMF exposure, I challenge you to out it to the test and see if it makes a difference in your day to day and how you feel.

Cold Showers

———

Contribution from Timbrey Lind,
RDH

A routine cold shower can do wonders for the health of your body and mind. The most important one that stands out to me, is it has a direct effect on our mitochondria, which is the powerhouse of our cellular system. Its primary function is to create energy and the cold resets the mitochondria or wakes it up in a way.

Another benefit - it reduces stress levels. Taking cold showers imposes a small amount of stress on the body, which leads to a process called hardening. This means that your nervous system gradually gets used to handling moderate levels of stress. This can help you handle stressful situations better.

It creates a higher level of alertness by waking your body up. It stimulates you to take deeper breathes, decreasing the level of CO_2

throughout the body, helping you concentrate, keeping you more focused.

It contributes to a more robust immune system by increasing the amount of WBC's. These blood cells protect your system against diseases. This increases your metabolic rate, which stimulates the immune response.

Cold showers can help with weight loss because cold increases your metabolic rate, it also stimulates the generation of brown fat. Brown fat is a specific type of fat tissue that in turn generates energy by burning calories.

This is something that you can do every morning as a routine to start your day off. After a workout is another time that it is most beneficial. And if you are like me who cannot give up their hot showers, you can always end the shower in cold water for about 30 seconds to a minute and still get the benefits.

Grounding

———

Contribution from Timbrey Lind, RDH

Grounding is a practice that everyone should be doing.

It consists of walking barefoot on the ground and connecting with nature for 30 min a day. Sometimes your location is not conducive for grounding (winters in the north), so a grounding mat is another option as well.

When you put your feet to the ground, we are allowing the electrons that the ground has, to be absorbed through our body. It is like taking handfuls of antioxidants. It supports the organ system and the tissues specifically.

95% of people walk insulated on the earth. We wear shoes that completely disconnect us from being able absorb the electrons the earth offers us.

Grounding has a lot of benefits and yet, it is SO simple. Some of those benefits include reducing inflammation, lowering the stress response, improved sleep, reduced pain, increased cortisol release, enhances circadian rhythms, speeds healing, improves athletic performance, EMF mitigation and much more.

Grounding involves coupling your body to the earth's surface energies by walking barefoot or sitting outside.

When your body is inundated with these negative electrons abundantly present on the earth's surface, your body immediately equalizes to the same electric potential as the earth.

Grounding is free, but we are so rarely connected to the ground since we wear rubber sole shoes all day and live-in high-rise apartment complexes.

There have been a lot of studies done on "grounding" or "earthing". This is one way to relax into your parasympathetic state.

Burnout

—

I want to end this book with the topic of "burn out".

One definition of "Burnout" reads: "A state of emotional, physical, and mental exhaustion caused by excessive and prolonged stress. It occurs when you feel overwhelmed, emotionally drained, and unable to meet constant demands." Today, more than half of us report record levels of "burnout" and this is a result of our choices in how we are living. I hope that you can make better choices for yourself, improving your life quality and health.

I came across a book written by two sisters (Emily Nagoski, PHD and Amelia Nagoski, DMA), both coming from different backgrounds and techniques, called "Burnout: The secret to unlocking the stress cycle." Anxiety comes from the accumulation, day after day, of stress that never ends. Dealing with your stress is a separate process than dealing with the things that cause your stress.

According to the Nagoski sister, physical activity is the single most efficient strategy for dealing with the stress response. Additional measures you can take include the deep, slow, diaphragmatic breathing we have discussed. Also, a long mindful kiss or a twenty second hug. Connecting with other people is a fundamental need, sharing energy with others in a positive way. Everyone has a different level of connection that they require, and it can vary at different times in our lives, but the fundamental need for it is always still there to some degree. This can be having a positive relationship of many types - friends, family, partners, co-workers... someone or some people who provide us with positive energy and interactions. According to "Burnout" this type of relationship can fuel our body just as eating nutritious foods and taking deep breaths do.

Another topic they focus on is oscillating between work and rest. When we allow proper time for both work and rest, the quality of our work improves along with our health. Mental rest is needed for your brain to process the world. Rest does not have to be doing nothing - resting your mind can include getting bodily exercise.

This is called active rest. And then there's sleep - the quality and quantity need we covered earlier. How much rest is adequate? Science says 42% which is about ten hours out of every twenty-four. It does not have to be every day, but it's an average over time. We have established by now that stress is a physiologic function that impacts every system and function in our bodies. To keep all our systems in full working order, science is telling us we need to rest in some manner for an average of ten hours out of twenty-four. This can be with sleeping, stress-reducing conversation with your positive connections, exercise, meditation, relaxing activities such as coloring or even paying attention to your food while you are preparing it or eating it.

Breathing, exercise, proper rest, and getting out of your stress cycles - are you seeing a pattern yet? Take care of yourself.